MW01167125

# TWO

# SIDES

# TO A MAN

# TWO

# SIDES

# TO A MAN

## The Silent Battles of a Black Man

### O.Diaz

PUBLISHED BY: O.DIAZ

Copyright © 2022 - All rights reserved

No part of this book may be reproduced or used in any manner without the prior written permission from the copyright owner, except for the use of brief quotations in book reviews.

Disclaimer Notice
Please note the information contained within this book is for education purpose only. The reader acknowledges that the author is not engaged in the rendering of medical and professional advice. Please consult a licensed professional for medical advice.

By reading this book the reader agrees that under no circumstance is the author responsible for any loses, direct and indirect that incurred as a result of the information contained within this book including but not limited to errors, omissions and inaccuracies.

Contact: info@twosidestoaman.com
Website: https://www.twosidestoaman.com
Instagram: @twosidestoaman
Hashtag: #TSTAM

# DEDICATION

*To all the black men battling mental health in silence, this book is dedicated to you.*

# Contents

*Black men's emotional
wellbeing and mental health
is often minimalised*

# TWO SIDES TO A MAN

# 1. Introduction

What drove me to write two sides to a man? In all honesty, it's a book that has been frantic to touch the surface. The black man is the most emotionally and mentally neglected man in society.

From my experience, black men's emotional wellbeing and mental health is often minimalised. I witnessed the black men closest to me internalise many struggles, which they tried to "soldier through" instead of being granted the safe space to recognise and overcome them.

Growing up, books that specifically emphasised, acknowledged, and catered to black men's daily battles without sounding clinical were rare. I wanted to create a digestible book that highlights and bring awareness to the conflicts black men experience and their struggle to integrate fully into society and cope mentally. I want black men to feel seen, heard and understood.

I will not chasten myself for being amongst those who did not understand the mental health of black men enough to speak out on it. But, with personal experience, I must bring great awareness.

This book highlights the battles black men face in society and its impact on their mental health. It explores the hidden sides in our communities, institutions and homes and the façade black men presents to the world to survive.

Black men need a refuge for their emotional pain and suffering. Mental health is a critical but often neglected issue, especially among black men. As a result, the mental health of black men is often silenced. "Two Sides To A Man" examines the sensitive topics concerning the black male experience, such as race, toxic masculinity, abuse, toxic parenting, sexuality, and social pressures. Black men are taught to suffer in silence at the hands of their trauma; this practice must be abolished.

The aim of the book is to give black men the

voice to speak out about their internal struggles and not fall victim to the stigmatising concept of shame. I hope to provide relatable awareness and healing.

I want to diminish the narrative that black men must be strong all the time and hide their abuse, hardships, and shortcomings. We need to teach black men to recognise, welcome and overcome their daily struggles, not avoid them.

I wanted to maintain a serious viewpoint when discussing some of the mental health issues dear to me. I also hope you enjoy the comforting approach throughout.

# TWO SIDES TO A MAN

*The more we provide our minds with negative, dark thoughts, the more ill we become*

# TWO SIDES TO A MAN

# 2. Mental Body

> **To help the problem, first, understand it**

When we discuss the intricacy of our mental health, we often forget to magnify the "mental" body. When referring to our "mental" health, what exactly are we saying? So frequently, we throw around the word or base our definitions on our level of comprehension and run with it. We say, "I need to work on my mental health", then enter a state of being lost immediately afterwards. We have not understood the "mental" aspect itself and how to work it or apprehend it.

Let's first recognise that your "mental" body is the spinal cord of your most authentic self. This unseen version expresses itself as your concrete intelligence, your mind. We base a man's every action on the vehicle of his mind, subsequently causing men to seek that very thing, their mind. You often hear successful men say, "now that I'm rich, I'm still so unhappy, I still get dark thoughts". They never seem to understand why their physical happiness is not manifesting into their mental state of being. They fail to acknowledge that striving for only physical contentment and neglecting their mental development hinders their true, complete happiness.

You must look after and develop your mind further than being sex centred, eating chicken wings, and drinking 1942. Develop your mental, emotional, psychological, and social intelligence.

The mind is a powerful vehicle that stores an infinite amount of data, including your memory, trauma, pain, imagination, and many more. Your mind can be your friend or your worst enemy.

Imagine a friend who knows all your deepest darkest secrets and uses them against you? It's like picking up a dagger and stabbing yourself in the back. Unfortunately, that is the reality of not conquering your mental body.

The mind has a funny way of magnifying your

trauma if you don't get to grips with it and control it. Have you observed when you're all alone at night, your most profound thoughts come alive? Once you enter a phase of being still, you enter a space of being more knowledgeable and able to take on any task. This occurrence can manifest as an outburst of creativity or a sudden gush of ideas for some people. For others, this can also cause their mind to race into overdrive and process every trauma, fear, and self-doubt in one sitting.

## You can control your thoughts

You're probably wondering, "well, how do I conquer my mind" or "how do I control which thoughts will arise". Your mind is your excellent servant. You must train it. Your mind knows no data other than what you store inside it. If you tell your mind you're worthless, it will register and store that data and amplify it times infinity.

Alternatively, if you tell your mind, you can conquer all; it'll unquestionably believe that too.

## Delusion is the key to success

Have you ever wondered why some of the most powerful men all had one thing in common? self-belief. So much belief it comes across as delusional. Self-belief refers to the "belief of their mind", "belief of the power their mind possesses". Self-belief is no delusion, I tell you. It's the art of training your mind to understand your power and programming your mind only to know your capabilities and not your shortcomings. If I'm honest, I believe a good dash of delusion is the key to abundant bliss.

Ceasing permission for your mind to store dark thoughts is like creating a paradise for yourself. Being delusional is great because it means you don't need to think about what areas you're lacking in, because you already believe you have excelled.

Unfortunately, we spoon feed our minds with negative thoughts so often that it consumes us and takes our minds into a state of arrest. The more we provide our minds with negative, dark thoughts, the more ill we become. Feeding the mind with negative thoughts is like poison, thus causing some to spiral into mental illnesses including depression.

When we discuss "mental" health, this is usually in reference to a man's ability to handle critical human functions, such as the ability to think, feel, express, and manage a range of both positive and negative emotions. It also refers to sustaining healthy, good relationships with others.

Commonly, black men believe the further they detach from their mental and emotional state of being, the better their mental health will be/become.

> Running from your problems
> is a race you will never win

We spend all our lives conjuring up new ways to pretend we don't care about our problems and try to suppress them. When really, you should be confronting them so you can truly free yourself. The very thing you are running from is already stored in your mind indefinitely and rears its ugly head when least expected if you don't face them.

Have you ever been sitting down and randomly had a thought about something you went through years ago that you thought you had put to the "back of your mind"? I bet you have. Now you're sitting at your work desk in excruciating torment out of thin air. You cannot physically suppress your thoughts or put them at the "back of your mind" because your thoughts are not tangible.

Therefore, adopting a suppressive coping mechanism will only cause your emotions to flare up in more negative ways in the relationship you have with yourself and with others.

- Confront your negative thoughts and challenge them with a positive way of thinking.

- When presented with negative scenarios, train your mind to only consume and energise what you instruct. You are the boss.

# TWO SIDES TO A MAN

*Systematic racism has a collective knock-on effect that slowly eats away at a black man's mental health*

# TWO SIDES TO A MAN

# 3. Systematic Racism

We are tired of educating and explaining to white people about racism. When the topic of racism comes up, everyone seems to sigh, huff and puff. We're all so exhausted by the wounds of racism that we've began to despise discussing it. It's like "ah not this again" a constant Deja Vu.

However, racism plays a contributing factor to a black man's mental health struggles, its simply ignorant to deny it's significance.

Evidence shows that black men are significantly more likely than other races to be diagnosed with severe mental health disorders and be sectioned under the mental health act. We must ask a prevailing and appropriate question, what do black men experience in the psyche when striving to survive and thrive in society?

When engaging in philosophical conversations with my black male friends, the common denominating factor affecting their mental health has been systematic racism, which has been persistent and profound. For those of you who are new to the concept of systematic racism, also known as institutional racism, it is a form of racism embedded in the laws and the regulations of a society or an organisation. This includes education, employment, housing, healthcare, and political representation.

Ironically, as a black man, you are expected to be the backbone of the community whilst facing the crippling barrier of this historic plague. Black men want the opportunity to flourish without firmly being tied to the hands of systematic racism, reducing the likelihood to access high earning jobs.

With the current unemployment rate higher for black men, drowning in the deep end is familiar and reoccurring. We know good formal education is an important factor of an individual's earning potential. However black boys are unlikely to continue to higher education due to the following reasons:

- Black boys are likely to receive harsher punishment in school than other groups.
- Black boys are not reading at a satisfactory level.
- Black boys are likely to be placed in special education programmes.

Black men unemployment rate is also higher for those minted out of graduate school than other demographics. This leaves them strapped with debt and frustrated about the high earning jobs that did not materialize.

The small percentage of black men that "make it" are idolised as the Greek Gods of society, a rare commodity. These men are hailed the 'knights in shining armour of the community.

All black men deserve fair opportunities to live without being regulated to an existence solely based on poverty, madness, and mayhem.

The male nature is full of pride, ego and outward chest. What man wants to feel less than his peers and underperforming in society? Being black does not change this.

> A Lion is an emblem of the dream of absolute power, he belongs to a world outside the realm of society and culture.

Like a lion, the epiphany of a black man is power and freedom. It's what gives the feeling of purpose. A Lion will go out and hunt its prey(money) and provide for its lioness(women) and cubs(children) whilst protecting its territory(home). All of which he gets to do with no limitations.

A black man's nature is to do the same. Lions

are the pride male. If we observe the elements of wildlife, females are attracted to power, strength, protection, and the ability to provide. All of which are evident in women of today.

The institutional construct denies black men the opportunity to earn fair wages which contributes to black families remaining below the poverty line. This unfair treatment continues the vicious cycle of poverty for black boys and men. Black men want more than just the ability to survive in society; they want the opportunity to thrive.

Suppose you're wondering why I previously used the analogy of the Lion in the wildlife, it highlights that black men are not particularly in the wild, but are bound to the jungle of society, whilst simultaneously being limited access to the resources to succeed.

Let's not pretend financial status isn't used to determine a man's societal value today. Therefore, black men having limited access to financial opportunities keeps them as the least valued men in society. Almost every black man I know has compared this discrimination to "feeling like there is no way out. Almost like you're stuck, or like you're reading a heroic book about yourself, and all the pages are missing."

Having a burning desire to win is great, but how does one win a game they are not allowed to play?

We undermine how this has played a considerable role in the mental health of black men and how they perceive themselves. The standard and value you hold yourself can feel like it has been majorly compromised.

Let's also explore when black men are granted the opportunity to be in spaces to make a good income. The settlement is usually to present a watered-down version of themselves to appear more digestible. You know? Less aggressive or intimidating to other counterparts merely for just existing.

How does one work in an environment putting

on a hat of a character they have never seen before? What happens if he mistakenly comes out of character? Will he be sacked? More times than none, the answer is yes. Now, what do you think that does to a black man's self-esteem? How does a black man maintain his confidence when he must alter himself to be accepted as well as tied to the shackles of submitting to another man? After a substantial amount of time, this will change how he views himself.

In my years of working in corporate settings, I watched many young, charismatic, "pep in their step" black men walk through the door, ready to take on the world. These men are often in their early twenties, you know, the age you believed the world was your oyster before you learned about oppression. But, after some time, I will notice these young black men leave the office looking beat down with their heads to the ground.

I'd also observe how much softer their voice got and how much it lost it assertiveness. Funnily enough, men of other races seemingly were still enjoying the privilege of being themselves or more pompous. I always found it unsettling how a black man feels he cannot be himself to be accepted. There is always the side he must present to the workforce and the side he can showcase in the comfort of an environment that truly serves him.

Why do so many black men want to work for themselves? Most have already encountered adverse experiences, which leads them to figure it out by themselves to avoid the Deja Vu.

# Systematic Racism Affects How Black Men Are Treated Under the Law

1 in 1,000 young black men are likely to be killed by the police in the U.S. We say "Fuck the police" so much it's become the national anthem. From

"thugs" to "hooligans:" the demonisation and criminalisation of black men is the real pandemic.

Being black is a synonym for crime in a racist society. Black men are seen as crazy, unhinged and a threat to society. They label black men thugs, but who are the real thugs? Black men are subjected to racial profiling, police brutality and are likely to be pulled over by the police when going home. So, we must ask the weighty question, what is the checklist for being a threat to society? Black?

Police exploit the negative stereotypes of black men being violent and dangerous as a method of imposing prejudice without consequence. Naturally, these encounters with the police and the ensuing stress can have negative effects on the black man's mental health. Almost all the black men I know from different education and social backgrounds have had an adverse experience with the police at some point in their lives.

Subsequently, most young black men from an early age do not trust the police and uphold the 'fuck the police' mentality. This is not out of rebellion, but for the unlawful, unjust, and misconduct from the police. Calling the police is like a death wish. You call on them and somehow, you're the villain. You are now incriminated for something you didn't do.

So, how does one traverse in areas that deny and hate him? Systematic racism has a collective knock-on effect that slowly eats away at a black man's mental health, self-esteem, and how he will perceive himself in society.

"Don't shrink yourself, surround yourself with those that think and **ink** like you"

*Rejection is redirection*

# TWO SIDES TO A MAN

# 4. Overcome Rejection

We all fear rejection. The only difference is that some admit it, and some don't. In a world where black men are often rejected in different capacities, the feeling of someone saying "no" to you can leave you feeling worthless, devalued, and unwanted. No matter who the "no" is coming from, we all believe we are worth something and that something should be valued across the board.

There are a series of ways men can experience rejection, be it a job, breakup, family members, friends. So, it's fair to say no matter the magnitude of the rejection; it still has an impact on your mental health.

When you think of rejection, you hardly consider how it progresses into feeling just as painful as being kicked in the nuts.

Rejection has a way of being so intense that it can have a negative effect on your mental health. I mean, the human mind is vulnerable to main character syndrome after all, so why would it believe it could possibly be rejected. So, when faced with rejection, the emotions that come with it can create a sense of low self-esteem, anger, sadness, and the feeling of a bullet to the chest.

As we know, black men deal with rejection on many different frequencies; let's take institutionally, for example. You have polished and prep for an interview that you're more than qualified just to be dismissed within the first ten minutes of walking in solely for the elephant in the room, your skin colour. The feeling of walking out of the interview knowing you've been rejected because of something completely out of your control can cause a series of negative emotions and anger. So how do black men avoid getting rejected in a world that rejects men like him every day?

There are, of course, more common instances of rejection for men, such as the painful scorn of a woman. The burning desire to speak to a woman you have been eyeing at the coffee shop every morning, you take the leap of faith, but she utters those three magic words, "I'm not interested". This can cause an instant series of racing emotions. Feeling angry, hurt, embarrassed and instantly feeling a sense of worthlessness. This, for you, feels like the icing on the cake to all the problems you're already suppressing.

We must note it's perfectly normal to feel let down and a gust of sadness when experiencing rejection. Still, you must first recognise you do not need to take refuge in this place of pain. Then, you can recognise it's not about you and free yourself.

Black men hate to admit some of their greatest fears stem from the fear of rejection. This fear derives from being unable to process the feeling of being rejected, usually because they cannot handle the emotions that come with it. In a world where black men commonly conceal their emotions, rejection is like the broom that sweeps it to the surface. Rejection would mean they would have to confront self-doubt and, God forbid, confronting insecurities. Owning up to having insecurities to a man is like stripping him of his secure-male badge of honour. We all know how hard men find it to admit to having insecurities, but the reality is we all do. If we didn't, rejection wouldn't feel so unbearable

Some black men have adopted the "not trying at all" stance in hopes it will save them from the gruesome wound of rejection. Subsequently leading them to miss out on opportunities that would have embraced them. Ever heard, "you miss 100% of the shots you don't take" well, this is true.

If we consume ourselves with the fear of rejection, the likelihood is it controls us. What you fear controls you and every decision you make. The fear of rejection causes you to not take risks, and we know the secret ingredient to success is risk-taking. Right? Does accepting rejection mean you will win all the time? No. Does it mean you will be embraced in every room you walk into? No. But dammit, it means whether you win or lose, you still maintain the same confidence and self-esteem you came in with.

Now, I can unpack how the effects of rejection has affected black men's mental health for hours, but instead, I want to get black men to a place where rejection can be endured, and the quality of life still feels abundant.

## Get rid of your entitlement

Yes, as hard as it is to fathom, it is not always about you. More times than none, rejection has more to do with the other person than you. We must recognise every human being is operating from a place of their perception of the world, which they are entitled to and if you do not fit their fantasy, you will be rejected. Similarly, if they don't fit yours, you will reject them. You both possess the same power in the draft for what you are looking for.

In the cases where race is involved black men, if you are rejected due to prejudice, you must understand this is not your load to carry. It has everything to do with the offender, their perception of life and their way of thinking. Their internalised racism is something you cannot relate to, and rejection, in this case, is a florescent angel saving you from hell.

## Avoid negative thoughts about yourself

When dealing with rejection, it's easy for our minds to trace back to every possible slavery scenario and wonder why we must suffer so much as black people. It's easy to believe rejection is a personal attack on us. Rejection leaves you wondering whether you are good enough, worthy and deserving of love. When rejected, we dissect every aspect of ourselves and label them undesirable. We now question ourselves, our capabilities, our appearance, our character and try to summarise ways to "fix" the parts of us we believe were the cause of the rejection. Black men quietly fall victim to this.

I want you to understand all of this is counterproductive. Give yourself a break. Recognise none of this is what your mind needs to process rejection; this just further fuels insecurity. Ultimately, you will never know what someone truly wants in a partner, employee, friend etc., so how can we replicate it? Instead, give yourself kind words, affirming words that you are good enough, instead of crippling yourself with negative thoughts.

## Ride the emotions

So, you've been rejected, and you're feeling hysterical. Give yourself permission to feel these feelings. Give yourself the grace to discern these feelings are completely normal and nothing to be ashamed of. Even if it means taking an hour or a day to completely process the rejection, so be it. Avoid minimalising your emotions; deal with them headfirst to avoid them re-emerging at a later stage.

## Grieving the loss of the expectation

When we think of grief, we forget to recognise grief comes in many forms, expectations, dreams and longings. They provide us with hope and motivation in some cases, but when they are not attained, they can break our spirit, question ourselves, purpose and contentment. So, grieve the expectation that you weren't chosen and allow yourself to experience these stages without shame.

# Avoid lashing out

When rejected, it can easily trigger emotions of abandonment or neglect. These feelings can stir up a vast range of aggressive emotions if not tamed. Life is full of rejection, we can't win all the time, so if we do not deal with our internal triggers surrounding rejection, every time you're rejected will send you into a cardiac state.

The thing about rejection is you have no control over the person doing it. We all know men like to have a reasonable amount of control in their lives, so when presented with something you can't control, it can leave you feeling powerless. And if not controlled can cause you to want to lash out.

Feeling overwhelmed is okay, but how we convey our emotions is where we need to be careful. Instead of projecting your internal triggers, process rejection as part of life. It builds character. Discern you aren't the first to be rejected and certainly will not be the last.

*Rejection is a common occurrence. Learning that early and often will help you build up the tolerance and resistance to keep going and keep trying. - Kevin Feige*

*Heightism is the last unchecked prejudice.*

*Alice McDermott*

# TWO SIDES TO A MAN

# 5. Heightism Is Real

Let's not pretend a man's height has never been a discussion and deciding factor when determining his desirability today. Though it is discussed in private 'chats' or when a woman declares her "preference", we forget that this is an act of discrimination. Discriminating against a man solely based on his height is called "Heightism", and it is real.

Heightism relates to the unfair treatment based on height, including prejudice and discrimination against those of shorter stature. This phenomenon affects multiple aspects of life in contemporary society, men being the key sufferers.

When the ideal man is profiled, women are often relentless in expressing that he must be "tall, dark and handsome". Leaving shorter men, well, disqualified. So, although black men are faced with many definitive setbacks in society, we can't turn a blind eye to bodily related prejudice, heightism.

You hear black women say all the time, "I don't know why this short guy thinks he can speak to me" or "men under 6 foot are my little sisters". As ignorant as these sentiments are, this is the common consensus of many black women today. What is ironic is that these statements are projected by women on what I like to say, the shorter side. Suggesting a man is simply not a "real man" if he is not six feet is absurd.

I won't say black women are all to blame for fuelling this stigma. I believe the media perpetuates these stereotypes too. Let's look at modern TV shows. How many times do we see a lead black woman having romantic relationships with a shorter man? Yet, we see plenty of tall men relationships with very short women. Still, the response is often very different come hell or high water.

I mean, of course, the only exception to seeing a woman with a shorter man is if he was a man of a substantial amount of wealth. Moreover, numerous social surveys have concluded the role of mass attitudes in the institutional privileging of tall people.

In men, the public conjured many bias-related arguments correlating tallness to positive attributes such as intelligence, masculinity, dependability, and leadership. Consequently, leaving shorter men feeling alienated in society. What is incredibly interesting to me, according to author Arianne Cohen of "The Tall Book", men that are taller get promoted more, paid more and considered in a better position to lead as opposed to their shorter counterparts. Not because they are more qualified, but simply for possessing more "socially attractive" attributes.

Whenever I have spoken with shorter male friends, they have confessed that they are often conscious of their height and ability to speak with women. "When I would message a woman on Instagram, my first question would always be how tall are you so I could quickly discern when to exit, without facing rejection". This results in toxic male stereotypes that continue to multiply in society. You would often hear black women tease that a black man had "short man syndrome", which further amplifies the decline in black men's mental welfare.

The oppression of being short is in line with the myths surrounding tallness. So, does this mean that women cannot be discriminated against, of course not. However, society identifies tallness as an attribute reserved for men.

Society must stop setting "normal" superficial standards for something out of men's control. Height isn't something you can wake up one day and determine whether you want to be short or tall; the discriminatory, prejudicial treatments stemming from heightism is outrageous. We don't emphasise enough how "ideal attractive attributes" like heightism has constantly been unattainable and has led many to suffer through anxiety, depression, low self-esteem, eating disorders and even suicide.

Some may configure bias against short men as just humour or non-existent, but this is the reality for many. black men. I want you to understand your experiences with heightism are real and valid. The effect of heightism culminates in irreversible damage and trauma to one's mental health. We must ask ourselves why we are more concerned with the appearance of a man than his mental health? A lifetime of feeling alienated in society is more crucial than any 'aesthetic'.

We need to first conjure up what it truly means to be a man. Something as superficial as a man's structure in measuring his masculinity is one of the problematic practices we must unlearn in the black community.

Abolish "short man syndrome" or referring to short men as "sis". Witty or not, these are very damaging. I want black men to understand your masculinity is not measured by your height or any physical attribute you possess, short or tall.

Your character, accomplishments, intelligence and wisdom will give you more power in every room than being just 'tall' can. We must aid black mental health by removing height hierarchy and conventional stereotypes to allow black men to take ownership of their masculinity and feel worthy, valid, and desirable just the way they are.

*Focus on important attributes that do not go out of fashion, like character, which cannot be replicated*

# TWO SIDES TO A MAN

# 6. Comparison Is the Thief of Joy

Everyone compares themselves to others at some stage in their lives; it is human nature. Therefore, suggesting one should never compare themselves to others is simply unrealistic. However, when we start doubting our abilities, that's when Houston we have a problem. Admiration is a beautiful thing, including amongst men, but it should not hold power to alter the quality of life.

Social media has made it borderline impossible to escape the exposure of witnessing successful black men in the media, be it musicians, athletes, or crypto gods, thus making you substantially more prone to comparing yourself to these men. Women flock to these men at the whim, cuban link chains and don't let me forget, the state-of-the-art sport cars. Black men are left wondering how they will live up to these seemingly unattainable standards.

The black community is just a fraction of the population. It borderline impossible to thrive in a society that has made black men more vulnerable to what I like to call "invisible competition". Invisible competition refers to men' pinning' themselves up against other men in their minds, torturing themselves with their shortcomings and subsequently damaging their mental health.

With the percentage of black men who manage to overcome poverty and make it lower than other demographics, the lengths black men will go to win by any means steals their true joy. Spending a lot of your time keeping up with other men to ensure you are ahead and not underperforming steals away true satisfaction with your own life. These unhealthy lengths to measure your success in life only causes stress, anxiety, and depression.

Instead, find joy in your process and purpose. Comparison is the biggest thief of joy, and black men are frequent victims of this. Though men refuse to admit it, they want to be the man other men want to be like.

## "Don't try to impress other men"

Many times, I'd hear the men around me saying "bro, did you see that Amiri shirt he had on, watch me get something better and really show them". It's funny, because I'd watch them go through great lengths to be in competition with one another, unprovoked.

• Purchasing expensive clothing items to mimic what is seen in the media rarely is to impress women; commonly, it's to impress other men during their "invisible competition" phase. Wanting to be the ultimate 'goat' is another real pandemic. There is no such thing, and you will tire yourself trying to compete to keep up. Sadly, black men are not granted the opportunity to win in white spaces, so they now invest their time competing with one another, wearing white-owned garments.

If you're honest with yourself, you don't want to really spend all that money on new designer shoes, it's just the pressure you've created to keep up with the latest trends that's consuming you. Let's face it, it's unhealthy to juxtapose yourself to the ever-changing ways of the world. Society's ideology of the perfect, cool, black male does not serve you; it is draining you financially and mentally.

I want black men to find contentment in themselves irrespective of what other black men are doing or, should I say, "pretending to be doing". You're not worthless because another man is driving a bigger car than you or has a bigger house. You'll realise the only person that truly cares about this is you.

I can assure you nobody wakes up in distress

because you're not a billionaire today. You're torturing yourself. Focus on important attributes that do not go out of fashion, like character, which cannot be replicated.

*Character is power — Booker T Washington.*

# TWO SIDES TO A MAN

*You can't wear a shoe that is not your size, nor can you wear a shoe that was tailored for someone else*

# TWO SIDES TO A MAN

# 7. Man Of the House

There is this historic tradition that has been moonwalking through black households and I'd like to take a moment to bring awareness to it. It's what I like to call the "Man of the house" complex. This refers to the unhealthy role young black males take on in replacement to absent fathers in the household.

I must add when I say 'absent' I'm also calling out the fathers that are physically present in homes, but provide no moral, financial or emotional support.

The lack of strong father figures is causing young black men to step up to the plate before they are mentally, physically, or emotionally ready for it. Not to mention the unhealthy relationships it causes between mother and son co-dependencies.

I always found it interesting how much black mothers have convinced themselves that its healthy for their adolescent sons to assume these destructive adult roles.

Black mothers have an intriguing way of deluding themselves into believing their sons cannot be overwhelmed or suffering internally attempting to live up to this phenomenon of the "man of the house".

Not only are young black men always referred to as the 'man of the house' when the fathers are not present, but they are expected to take on roles qualifying them for it. I have noticed a lot of black mothers are still grieving the loss of a solid two parent household and alternatively try to replicate it with their sons taking on the role of 'dad', both financially and emotionally.

This constant "adultification of childhood" where young black men are driven to adopt adult responsibilities prematurely has its own worries. Young men who are rising to the responsibility of being the man of the house is pressurising and damaging to their mental health.

Like I always say, "You can't wear a shoe that is not your size, nor can you wear a shoe that was tailored for someone else."

Dare I also mention how the implications of "man of the house" influences how black men navigate through society. The pressure to provide can nurture them into a life of crime. When young black men are unable to attain secured employment due to systemic racism and fewer opportunities to succeed legitimately, it's easy to take on the "by any means necessary mentality". If you're wondering what I mean by that, this mentality refers to choosing the easiest way of getting money, no matter what it takes. Usually, crime and violence.

When you have assumed the role of the provider of the house prematurely, it is hard for one to supress thoughts and actions of crime. Studies have shown that children growing up in intact married families are least likely to commit delinquent acts.

I truly believe this urban phenomenon we call man of the house has contributed to the black male repeated stressors. I've witnessed so much ownness on black males to save their mothers from the same poverty they have struggled to escape from. With the odds already stacked up against black males, the constant pressure to provide for their mothers, siblings as well as themselves is very crippling.

They feel the responsibility to fix all that is missing and all that is lost in crunching time frames. Not to mention how the glorification in the black community of becoming overnight millionaires to take our mothers 'out of the hood' generates unnecessary pressure and fuels this stigma. Young men feeling in debt to their mother is the real controversy. We never discuss how many black men take on the burden of carrying their entire family out of poverty because of being the man of the house. Which ironically ends up being the demise of their mental welfare.

There are many young men in our community playing the role of man of the house in their homes. I remember a conversation with a young man in his late teen whose experience is not rare. He came from a single parent household as his father was a violent alcoholic. As the only child he felt pressured to man up. His mother would often ask him to "be a man and bring us back some money, you can't just stay home, you need to help me out, you're a big boy now'.

He expressed his struggles of finding a job or other legitimate opportunities which caused him to have dark thoughts. He fell into crime to make money by any means necessary to provide for his mum and make her proud of him. However, he constantly feared he'd lose his life due to his gang affiliation. He often felt so drowned, overwhelmed he suffered from depression and PTSD. He ended up so manic he was worried she'd end up all alone, No Money, No Son. He explained there were times he felt so buried with the pressure he wanted to take his life. Sadly, he felt he couldn't share his mental state with his mother as he was also her emotional support.

My encounter with this young man flared my desire to shed light on the severity of the "man of the house" complex and how deep its chips into a black man's mental health and the complexities that still follow him into adulthood. The constant pressure to be the head of the house from a young age must be destroyed.

I truly believe young men should have the privilege to enjoy their youth without feeling in debt to family members. Being the man of the house should not be dignified at the detriment of your mental or physical wellbeing. Black mothers must rid themselves from these expectations of raising "manly boys" to provide for their home and recognise that their sons cannot be saviours to their struggles. Black mothers must also recognise their sons neglecting their mental health in return for riches is venomous. The feeling of not being a real man or inadequate is destructive. Not to mention how the elements of this complex chips away at men in adulthood, causing grown men to still feel in debt to their mothers or seek validation further down the line.

## "Don't try to be a hero"

Understand it's okay to not live up to this stereotype of the man of the house. As much as you may feel the ownness is on you, the reality is, it's not your responsibility to provide financial stability or emotional stability.

Most importantly do not let the pressures of poverty tempt you into a life of crime and shorten your lifeline. You must recognise you are your mother's son, not her saviour.

# TWO SIDES TO A MAN

*Young men must be taught from an early age to be aware of the ebbs and flows of mental health*

# TWO SIDES TO A MAN

# 8. Wooden Glasses

Let's not pretend it's easy to speak to black parents about your shortcomings. Discussing mental health in the black community is nothing short of a "taboo" or the elephant in the room. So much that black parents deny their sons the privilege of speaking about their mental welfare. I consider it the "wooden glasses" complex. An urban phenomenon of black parents putting on opaque glasses to blind themselves from reality concerning mental health.

Oh, how the "hush hush" method has always been implemented among us. As a matter of fact, it is considered "dirty laundry" of some sort.

There seems to be initial shame when discussing the mental wellbeing of their sons with "oh he just likes being in his room for days on end" or "he just behaves like that, don't worry about him", with usually no follow up action or thought on why that is.

It's often swept under the rug in fears of confronting it themselves. They know there is a problem, but they hope if they avoid it long enough, it'll somehow go away.

Black parents are extremely proud and boastful due to their own struggles and see their sons as a trophy that signifies their accomplishments.

> ## "Black parents have contributed to the problem"

As much as we hate to admit it, our caring parents are more consumed with how it would look on them than the turmoil their sons are going through. I strongly believe our parents have not tended to acknowledge their children's mental health because they have yet to challenge their own.

Our parents and parent parents have endured

years of racism, abuse and trauma and have the same mentality of "I went through this when I was your age, and I'm still alive, aren't I"?

Black parents glorify the struggle, usually because their parents glorified it too, it was all they ever knew. There was never room or space to discuss how the struggle impacted their mental health. Their coping mechanism was to just plough through it and come out the other end alive.

The black community glorify the struggle so much that we neglect our mental health in the process. In fact, the struggle should bring us closer to an atmosphere of openness and awareness. Our parents should pass down healthy coping mechanisms from their experience instead of sweeping them under the rug.

Young men must be taught from an early age to be aware of the ebbs and flows of mental health, should they not? It shouldn't be a case of "he's too young to understand" or "he's just isolating himself as teenagers do" or "don't mind him, he just likes to ignore everybody sometimes".

As sad as it is to admit, most black boys can't speak to their parents about anything they experience due to either being belittled or it subsequently ending in a lecture or brawl. (literally). Talking to your parents about anything remotely emotion-driven was like talking to a brick wall, a sturdy one at that.

> "Emotional negligence, is not emotional intelligence"

Black parents have a history of building a divide between themselves and their children in hopes to preserve the "respect". This causes them to have no idea on earth the mental torments their sons are going through. I always found it ironic how many black males were exposed to gang violence, drugs, and crime yet somehow, their parents didn't have a clue. Unless, of course, they had completely gone off the grid or violently harmed. this is the common emotional neglect black parents engage in.

Instead of being checked up on, black sons are usually left to it, unless it's regarding education or somewhat. There is a level of denial black parents hold, so I refer to it as a wooden glasses complex. Once they put these daily 'wooden glasses' on, it provides them the facade of ignorance to the mental health of their children.

I also question whether black parents put on these wooden glasses to hide from the reality of it or they genuinely do not have the correct guidance to address and provide the right support. Parents must look for changes in their son's behaviour and have open and honest conversations about their mental health. I urge all black parents to tend to the mental and emotional needs of their sons. This does not ruin your image, it protects it. Communicating with your children does not alter the respect. It gives you enough insight to raise the best. Afterall, what glory is a parent that neglected their child in times of need?

Battling with your mental health is hard enough, but to be faced with parents who will advocate for you "manning up" on top is the icing on the cake. I know sometimes you feel alone, and you can't share an ounce of weakness with those closest to you. But I will always say, find it within your hearts to understand your parents are unable to tend to your mental needs because they haven't managed to conquer theirs. Our parents could be fighting their own demons.

So, avoid isolating yourself because your family have the inability to aid your pain. Understand even if they did, they are not licensed doctors or therapists. Open your hearts to receiving therapy without shame or guilt.

*Every human being in society has the right to deny sex at any stage, male or female, irrespective of the sexual stereotype*

# TWO SIDES TO A MAN

# 9. Sexual Abuse

Society is so conformed to the ideology of black males being sexually aggressive and violently aggressive that the concept of them being victims has been displaced. Black males are not considered or researched enough as victims of sexual violations. Instead, black males are deemed only to be predators and perpetrators of sexually violent acts.

Black boys have been vulnerable to sexual predatory by older women, as research has shown, yet somehow, this is often silenced. The vulgar way males are viewed sexually feeds the stigma that they cannot be victims. Black men are perceived as hypersexual beings, leading society to believe they can never say "no" to sexual conquests.

The misconception that only women can be sexually abused is damaging to the black community and the mental health of black men and young boys. This stigmatisation does not urge young black men to come forward and speak out on the matters surrounding their sexual abuse. You often hear unwarranted bias arguments suggesting black men "simply cannot be raped or abused," which is completely absurd. Every human being in society has the right to deny sex at any stage, male or female, irrespective of the sexual stereotypes.

Society is so accustomed to categorising black men as predators that they somehow overlook how many women have sexually abused infants, boys, and men. Being a predator is not 'gender' exclusive.

Black males do not want to be exploited in the name of sexuality or your idea of how they should experience sex. An outstanding number of black males are survivors of childhood trauma of sexual abuse. These males have buried their trauma in hopes of it 'going away' because they are aware of the way current society undermines their trauma surrounding sexual abuse.

Black men should not be taunted with the idea

that they can only propose sex and never refuse it, especially when many of the abused males are infants and young boys.

## "Black males can deny sex"

I always found it unsettling the number of black males who lost their virginity to women double their age. They also didn't realise it was grooming and predatory until they were older, leading to a range of emotions.

We must abolish the "shut up and put up" stance surrounding black trauma as a black community. This unhealthy way of coping and keeping trauma inside the family instead of speaking with a therapist is poison to the soul.

Black men who experienced sexual abuse often feel they cannot open up to their confidants about their sexual abuse due to fear of not being perceived as "masculine" since society has proven time and time again to dehumanise their trauma and invalidate their emotions. As a community, we should spend more effort creating charities for black male survivors of sexual abuse and aid their mental health.

I want black men to know their experiences and trauma surrounding sexual abuse is real and valid. Your experience of trauma, pain and exploitation is not less significant because you are a male. Your eligibility to manhood is not compromised because of your sexual trauma. Your voice is seen, felt and matters.

*Men usually prefer to not speak on sexual pressures because it's a blow to the below*

# TWO SIDES TO A MAN

# 10.  Sexual Pressures

You're probably wondering what sexual pressures has to do with the mental health of black men or how the two coincide. Men feel the pressure to please their partner, and feel secure in their ability to perform sexually.

You often notice that young men are more open to exploring their sexuality early and understanding their bodies. They become inquisitive and want to explore and interact with various aspects of sexuality.

We're all very aware that come a certain age; young men become eager to explore themselves sexually by masturbation, having sexual partners or even comparing genital size in the locker room, typical boy behaviour. However, we don't emphasise the negative effects this may have.

A large group of black men suffer from 'size dysmorphia'. Meaning they experience a state of unhappiness and dissatisfaction with their penis size. With urban myths suggesting black men have the largest penises in humanity, this leaves those that do not fall under the category feeling inadequate and self-conscious. The emphasis on black men living up to the big penis stereotype, has had a negative effect on many black males' mental health. In reality a lot of women are more than content with any penis size, they also just felt peer pressured to adhere to liking these standards. So, in conclusion, we're all just living one big, fat lie. Nevertheless, we must recognise body dysmorphia is not exclusive to women, black men experience it too.

There are also other sexual pressures black men face such as premature ejaculation, performance anxiety and erectile dysfunction. There is already pressure on men to overperform sexually and please their partner as a token of manhood. The flipside to this is how one perceives themselves if one is unable to do these things due to sexual problems, anxiety or insecurity. We already know a lot of how men view themselves directly correlates to how others view them, especially women.

Although sexual health is essential to overall health and wellbeing, it's so common for the health care side of sex to be overlooked. It's been estimated that over 150 million men suffer from erectile dysfunction, and the figure will increase beyond 322 million by the year 2025. Men tend to get macho or dismiss any conversation, pertaining to opening the file to discuss their "man downstairs". Of course, we know this stems from how the male sex organ is viewed and considered as a barometer for his overall manly essence. Impotence is considered a shock to the penis.

Men usually prefer to not speak on this because they believe it's a blow to the below and an outright evasion of their manhood. I feel the space to make an uncomfortable, squirmy topic comfortable needs to be normalised opening up without fear of their man card being revoked.

When we're talking black men, another force that must be considered is how often black men are cautious with who gets to discuss their sexual rendezvous. So, although the percentage of black people in the Uk is 3% and in the US is 13%. The percentage of Black doctors falls at 4% in the US and UK.

Erectile dysfunction is a serious issue and nothing to be ashamed of. It Is also very highlighted to your woman when she is ready to get some action; what will you say? Will you continue to hide or play the "I'm asleep card?" There's only so long it can be hidden for; this is why we must make it normal to discuss these matters and get the treatment to aid the erection.

I encourage all black men to not shy away from any sexual complications faced, find comfort in knowing women secretly go through just as many squirmy sexual complications as you, if not more.

A few years ago, my male friend suffered from severe depression; when a psychologist spoke with him, she discussed some of the complexities he faced. I remember him mentioning that he struggled with erectile dysfunction as a teen, which caused him to suffer low self-esteem, subsequently causing him to sink deeper into depression. The irrational fear of not being able to perform sexually, have a girlfriend, a family of his own one day if he didn't manage to fight this problem, consumed him. The paradox was he is an overachiever, always did very well academically and is very handsome. Some would think there is no possible way a man of his calibre couldn't perform sexually, which is the reality for some young black men.

The feeling of worthlessness caused him to have no sexual desire or self-esteem communicating with women, plummeting him deeper into depression. A lot of black men struggle to come forward about issues that pertain to their sexuality or sexual abilities.

When my male friend opened up to his dad about his ED, to no surprise, his dad's first response was, "you're just shy, son. Do I need to bring some strippers for you or something"?

This is the common sarky responses given to black men when they attempt to open up. Black men are almost not allowed to fall short sexually without being teased. Another reason which causes them to suffer in silence. Why is he not immediately offered the specialist help from a professional? Why must he be mocked before he is helped? Black men are taught that even their sexual ability can be shamed, whilst women are granted compassion in this area.

"If boys don't learn, men won't know", as quoted by Douglas Wilson. So, it's important that we enforce these same methodologies as a community, raising strong black men, not by physique, but of emotional intelligence. Teach them to find safety in expressing their struggles.

The inability to live up to societies sexual

ideology of the black male does not define manhood.

# TWO SIDES TO A MAN

*Breaking up and breaking down is the common way black men cope with their mental health in relationships*

# TWO SIDES TO A MAN

## 11.   The Silent Killer of Relationships

We are facing a real psychological epidemic, the practice of pretending not to care, and it's spreading fast. The belief that one can simply supress and avoid their emotional and mental misfortune instead of confronting them is a real crisis.

Black men have opted for the dominant culture of toxic masculinity. The concept of the "oh so profitable" "manhood" continues to create a narrative that teaches men that suppressing their conscience is necessary to survive. Consequently, causing a disconnect in their relationships.

Emotional vulnerability is a fundamental resource of black men's emotional wellbeing and mental health. Therefore, shouldn't this vital piece of information be stored in a trophy cabinet upstairs? Unfortunately, young black men are taught to disown, reject, and avoid this natural emotion.

Emotional intelligence has been found to serve as the shield against depression and suicide. In addition, studies have shown that being open about one's emotional troubles is therapeutic in itself. Black men are so accustomed to putting their woman's emotions first they have sadly managed to neglect their own. In any healthy relationship both parties emotions and mental health is significant, there is no hierarchy.

# There's no such thing as a 'real man'

Many black men have admitted that devaluing vulnerability has hindered their emotional growth. The unhealthy connotation that to be a "real man", one mustn't acknowledge emotional turbulence such as fear, pain and sadness, is misery attempting to govern our culture. The glorification of hypermasculinity has voided the ability to create deep, personal connections and relationships with women and others.

Okay, fine, we won't pretend society doesn't ridicule black men for being emotionally vulnerable only to resent them for not showing the very emotion which they told them to neglect.

When a black man is combatting mental health whilst in a relationship, the initial reaction is to ridicule him and deem him unlovable or emotionally unavailable. It's never, he has not been taught to show these healthy emotions and yes, he is still learning. Whether he is 21 or 41.

Let's look at some of the contributing factors why men associate showing emotion with weakness. Let's take a time machine all the way back to secondary school, shall we. Growing up, when a black boy shows an ounce of emotion to his girlfriend in the playgrounds, you'd often hear his friends tease or shame him. The taunting made it seem illegal for one to express themselves. It was categorised as being 'soft' and God forbid falling victim to that. Men grow up with the stigma that showing emotion, even towards a female, is something to be ashamed of, something that makes you weak. Why are black men shamed for showing healthy emotions in relationships instead of learning the skills to nurture and sustain them? The art of being able to express, feel and understand emotions contributes to your mental health. Companionship with a woman is a healthy part of life.

This practice of instructing young black men to become emotionally avoidant teaches them to not showcase any form of mental health distress to women to avoid appearing weak. This carries on in their adulthood relationships. But what do you think this does to a relationship?

When we think of the end of relationships, our initial thought is always infidelity or abuse. But we never stop to think of the silent killer of relationships, mental health. You see, mental health is not something you can physically see or touch. As a result, we underestimate the chaos it causes in matters of love. Mental illness is relentless when it chooses its victims, and it certainly doesn't take a back seat in the relationship either.

> "Vulnerability is not weakness; it is our greatest measure of courage"

Black men, how many times have you avoided opening up to your woman about your mental health in fear of appearing weak. Your childhood trauma now drives the narrative. How often have you become cold and distant instead of expressing your depression in relationships? Not because you didn't want to, but you simply have been programmed to believe being emotionally vulnerable is not an attribute of a "real man".

So now, you adopt a character of being emotionally distant in fear that your weakness will be preyed upon, the only way to protect yourself is to apply a guarded defence mechanism. You're afraid your shortcomings will be used as a dagger in times of despair. So, what do you do? You shut down completely and emotionally, causing a disconnect in your relationships.

Something I commonly hear black men say is, during their darkest times of mental crisis, their initial thought was to isolate themselves or, in many cases, completely sabotage the relationships instead of their mental health being exposed to a woman because "who wants to look weak".

Allowing toxic masculinity to drive you into emotional avoidance in your relationships is where the true troubles lie; Isn't manhood expressing oneself without fear?

'Breaking up and breaking down is the common way black men cope with their mental health without dealing with the exposure or extreme visibility from their partners. Feeling the need to conquer their mental health alone and combat it with isolation ironically feeds the problem further.

The idea that as men, you must be unemotional, dominant, and strong to be deemed a man irrespective of your mental state further fuels the toxic-masculinity plague that continues to shred through the black community. Feeling that you cannot express times of mental cripple, emotional anguish to sustain your validity in your gender must be abolished.

"Toxic Masculinity" is a social construct. Men who glorify this breed of masculinity to the detriment of their relationships with themselves and others suffer from their own internal insecurities. You are bigger than your masculinity. Recognise you do not need to be strong all the time. You're allowed to feel things and express emotions without fear. Your relationship should feel like your haven, a space to express yourself. Unlearn the unhealthy pattern of secluding yourself in hopes to eliminate the shame of your mental health or emotional state.

I know as men, you perceive yourselves as the heroic character, with the leather cape on that saves the damsel in distress, so feeling like the damsel can be a bit uncomfortable. But please recognise, in healthy relationships with women, you do not need to be the hero all the time; you're allowed to have moments of weakness.

Give yourself permission to feel depressed, give yourself permission to feel weak, give yourself permission to feel pain. Extend yourself grace in your relationships and stop silencing yourselves in fear of losing your black belt of manhood.

*"I cry a lot, but to admit it – de la soul (2001) "*

*Black men experience a vast range of mental health issues but are not allowed compassion or acknowledgement*

# TWO SIDES TO A MAN

# 12.    Trauma & PTSD

So many black men hear the words Trauma and PTSD and immediately say to themselves "nope, that doesn't apply to me" and resume suffering in silence. Black men are more prone to this denial.

As a community, we do not emphasise the ever-growing rate of black male trauma sufferers and how significantly less likely they are to come forward to utilise the mental health services. This stems from the negative stigma attached to it.

This issue particularly sparks me as my brother suffered a severe traumatic breakdown in his late teens because of PTSD. He began to experience an overwhelming personality change and became very irritable. He experienced sleep paralysis and sleep terrors. My bedroom was right next door to his, so witnessing his distress was devastating. Although this is difficult to share, I want to bring awareness to this as mental health does not discriminate regardless of your social status and educational background. He experienced a series of mental breakdowns stemming from trauma and PTSD and coming from an African household, this was reduced to initially rebelling then being under "spiritual attack". After years of suffering, he was finally checked into a hospital and started therapy. My experience with my brother highlights how black men's mental health can deteriorate due to lack of awareness and education within the family.

Black men experience a vast range of mental health issues but are not shown the same compassion or acknowledgement. It is often seen as violent, untamed or a threat. Studies suggest that 56-74% of black males exposed to traumatic events will have an unmet need for mental health services. This substantial percentage should highlight the growing number of black males facing constant silent battles daily with mental health and are fighting the dark cloud over their heads. Mental illness shows itself in many ways, be it isolation or mania.

As a community, though we are not all licensed therapists or psychologists, shedding light on mental health disorders stemming from factors such as trauma, PTSD, illness, and abuse is imperative. However, when I say 'shedding light, I am not referring to just reposting a savvy quote preaching to "be kind always" but rather advocating for all black men not to shy away from getting therapy and counselling and utilising the mental health services offered to them.

Whenever I would speak to my black brothers regarding getting therapy, it is always frowned upon due to the stigma surrounding treatment in our community. Having access to therapy is deemed a luxury in other communities, a privilege to speak to someone about your darkest moments. I always found it crazy how we deny ourselves the comfort of doing the same.

I always use the witty analogy of "if your leg fell off at this very moment, would you be too ashamed to be taken to the hospital in the name of pride, or would you be desperate someone got you the help you needed?" Though this is an extreme case scenario, the answers I got back were always identical; you would want the help you need to survive, preserve yourself, and live.

Black men insist on treating mental pain as less damaging than physical pain when both are catastrophic. They have upheld the 'if it's not broke don't fix it' mentality due to believing pain can only be endured in the physical realm and not the mental which isn't the case.

Do not let the fear of appearing weak, getting help or unhealthy coping mechanism of having to be strong all the time deceive you.

This is completely off-topic, but this reminds me of the stereotype that black men are irrationally petrified of dentist and doctor appointments. I always found this so humorous yet very factual. I have seen the most muscular, hulk-like, strongest black men flinch at the whim of the idea of medical attention. The fear of getting help is usually equated to feeling emasculated for not being able to endure the pain on your own. There is also a mistrust for medical health providers, especially amongst black men, as historically black bodies and organs have been abused by science to conjure discoveries and experiments for diseases. This has contributed to the lack of trust to attain medical aid.

When black people often hear the word "trauma", they automatically associate it with war or assault. So, we skip past the undiagnosed trauma and PTSD we faced every day. For instance, for black men several parts of the day can be traumatic, resulting in PTSD and trauma going undiagnosed.

When I mention daily PTSD and trauma, this can include stop and searches by police, institutional racism, violence, and crime. We don't discuss enough the gut-wrenching feeling a black man feels when a police car drives past at night, or the sound of a loud bang causes you to flee without knowing the cause. These are all symptoms of trauma that are often overlooked and slowly form into mental illness.

According to Carla Manley, a clinical psychologist, the caveat of this is that mental illness like PTSD causes physical pain. Ranging of physical symptoms such as muscle tension, pain, headaches, and restlessness. The pain is not always just mental; it can transfer to your physical body. At this point, it is not something you can ignore or overlook.

I once worked with a man who was a victim of police brutality years ago. The police beat him so gruesomely that the scars are still engraved deep in his skin to this day. He experienced the police brutality overseas. The police accused him of looking like someone they had wanted for "fraud and smuggling drugs", or so they say. You would assume the police would do their checks before beating him black and blue, but that's not the reality for a black man. Unfortunately, it's usual protocol to impose violent acts on black men and deal with the consequences after.

The scars were just a fraction of the pain he endured. He also mentioned experiencing sleep terrors causing him to experience trauma flashbacks, nightmares, and poor sleeping experience. I was sympathetic and understood his suffering as my brother had experienced similar symptoms. I have become sensitive on matters of mental health and pick up on signs of flaring and active mental illness or people generally suffering in silence. Like many black men, he was carrying the weight of trauma on his shoulders and ashamed of the thought of opening up to anyone about his illness.

Black men are taught to uphold a mentality of being their brothers' keepers whilst in the same breath not trusting their brother enough to open up. As a result, they are left to harbour their struggles inside themselves.

Black men grow up with the mentality of not

trusting anyone, even themselves. There is no space to be open about their emotions or struggles. Nobody wants to feel emasculated within the social circle, so in return, nobody is willing to show their hand. Who does the black man turn to in times of emotional pain?

Unfortunately, this emotional suppression also replicated in our households. Let's go back to when we were merely kids. Daughters are usually allowed more grace for expressing emotions because it's a "girls thing". In contrast, a black boy coming of a certain age is laughed at or teased for even shedding a single tear.

Black men are taught to adopt the "strong" man mentality from an early age. They are trained to not show a fraction of hurt or upset as this was reserved for the "ladies". Young boys are antagonised for showing any form of hurt, pain or upset. Yet, we never discuss how these unhealthy coping mechanisms for emotional distress imposed on young black boys show up in darker ways in their adult life.

The unhealthy misconception that black boys are not allowed to cry is damaging. When raising your sons, teach them to be free, teach them to express healthy emotions, allow them to understand that emotions, pain and hurt are feelings to be explored, not suppressed. I always say it's always better to deal with the pain of today than the wound of tomorrow.

The minimalisation of mental illness around fellow black men is not uncommon either. Among friendships groups, I've witnessed men express going through a hard time and struggling with their mental state. It's often combatted with "come out for a drink, man, you need to be around some women, that's all" it usually never goes deeper than that. Honestly, I can't even say the friends are to blame. It's the blind leading the blind.

But let's be honest, how long can you use alcohol and women to mask the troubles you're facing? How long can you pretend that you're not drowning inside, feeling ill and destructing to protect your pride? After a while, it doesn't even feel the same. There's nothing like peace of mind. Therefore, it's imperative that we normalise getting specialist medical attention and not using avoidant coping mechanisms.

A famous quote from Jesse Owens once said, "the battles that count aren't the ones for gold medals. The struggles within yourself, the invisible battles inside us all, that's where it's at"

This quote particularly moved me because we often glorify the physical battles we can see, hardly the ones we're overcoming inside, like mental illness. The black community tend to only celebrate rising above the poverty line, buying a new house, car, or even that new diamond embezzled watch; believing those are the only accomplishments to be rewarded. Though these are tremendous assets, the greatest asset to glorify is the wellness of your mind. The real work is the preservation of your mental health. Conquering the battles we can't see, the invisible ones, the battles that truly deserve the trophies once they are overcome. The real prize is welcoming and expressing your mental health and freeing yourself from the stigmas of society.

We never discuss the power of welcoming and accepting our mental state, in whatever state it's in. Instead of beating ourselves down when we are struggling mentally, we should magnify it saying "I'm feeling terrible today, my mental health is at an all-time low. I accept it, and I'm going to get the help to overcome this" and doing just that.

Acceptance is freeing and allows room for help, healing, advice, and progression. Suppression teaches you to bear the burden of your troubles.

# TWO SIDES TO A MAN

*Sometimes it takes great suffering to pierce the soul and open it up to greatness"*

# TWO SIDES TO A MAN

# 13. The Power of Suffering

Suffering is not an unusual occurrence with black men. When faced with hard times, the initial thought is to beat yourself down, give up and feel helpless because you're taught there is no room for you to advance in this world. Black men are schooled to believe suffering is something to be ashamed of.

What if I told you there is power in suffering? Life is never easy and is a constant see-saw of lows and highs. Many humbling experiences will challenge you and try to break you down. Suffering is like batteries in your back that charge you up and make you stronger and wiser.

I've noticed the frequent demand black men are held, to always demonstrate ultimate strength and control during times of pain, sadness, anxiety, fear, suffering, and hurt. We live in a society now where ultimate self-control and emotional suppression, even in hard times, is rewarded, and acts of weakness are punished. Black men are left to sink to a place of isolation in fear of the perception of others, resulting in depression, anxiety, and addiction.

We should dignify the "power" of suffering when faced, because really who wants to win all the time anyway? Who wants to be happy all the time? You think you do, but how will you know happiness without sadness? Without losing, how will you know how it feels to win? See, when you suffer, it causes you to go deep inside yourself inwardly and confront the voices you've been running from; that is where you learn your true power and strength. There's usually no ego or pride in suffering; at this point, you are your truest self. The upside is when we are stripped of ego and pride, we have the ability to learn and overcome any obstacle. We mustn't consume our minds with negative thoughts in these moments because what you will learn is, the place of suffering you have been afraid of forces you to elevate to the next level of your being.

For all these years, we've been taught that there are consequences for losing and rewards for winning, but that's not always the case. There is, in fact, great power in suffering if you're patient enough to watch. Don't feel sorry for yourself, you're more powerful than you think. The world constantly imposes on us, "don't do this, do you want to end up suffering". "I hope I never have to suffer like him". I'm sure this sounds familiar to you. But what is suffering? Does the end result determine this?

Every day, you're torturing yourself with the imaginary fear that if you are suffering, it will last forever. You're falling victim to the fear that feeling forms of suffering equate to weakness or suffering is infinite. Black men constantly having to remain in a positive space all the time suggest black men being in "negative" space is something to be shamed, when instead we should dignify and overcome this.

# "You do not need to be happy all the time"

Black men do not need to constantly be in a positive space; only being positive has the ability to solely focus on your wins, which overshadows the process. We must teach black men that you can be both happy and sad; these are both healthy and normal emotions. So, when they are faced with times of suffering, they have the skills to conquer it and learn it's okay to not be okay.

During your times of suffering, you will notice you're more prone to focusing on the process, effort and areas of improvement. Suffering is not always easy but understanding that your hardships have the ability to make you smarter is imperative. Understanding the emotions during hardships also help you to build emotional intelligence and empathy.

When you are faced with something difficult, you are faced with tiny puzzles to solve. Such as how to save more money. For many black men, you never truly understood the value of money until you have finished splurging it all. Black men were never taught the value of financial literacy. Thus, landing them in a place of suffering. The upside is that suffering is a process that often can advance you to the next level of wisdom if utilised correctly. I'm not saying it's easy to suffer, but tough experiences are great cardio for the brain.

Sometimes, it is easy to panic during times of suffering and immerse your mind in negative thoughts. Black men are more prone to this due to their desire of being overcomers and overachievers. Suffering for black men can feel like being swallowed by a deep hole of quicksand.

Young men fantasise about a life full of riches, women and abundant happiness, so when confronted with times of suffering, it's easy to fall victim to the grief of your expectations. But how often do you hear success stories of men who did not suffer at some point? Suffering is part of the process and cannot be escaped in any capacity. In fact, successful, happy men praise their time of suffering. In life, we make this bargain all the time, trading pain for something better.

Studies have shown "post-traumatic growth", a phenomenon in which searching for good in major life crises results in psychological functioning and other mental health benefits. Therefore, it is important to stay level-headed during these moments; tough times do not last.

Hardships sharpen your emotional perceptiveness. During a tough time, you'll find yourself suddenly attracted to nature, animals, children playing and all sorts of Beethoven music. The human mind naturally submits to the natural attraction of life in the midst of its despair. A world full of beautiful things is a beautiful world, is it not? During hard times your mind now has the capabilities to process the things that truly matter.

In times of hardship, it helps make life feel richer in ways we once didn't appreciate. Sometimes, when chasing a world of material things, we land ourselves in dark spaces because they do not fulfil our inner desires. But during difficult times, we magnify the true beauty of life.

Do not be ashamed, Black man. In your times of suffering, understand this, *To live is to suffer, to survive is to find the meaning in the suffering – Friedrich Nietzsche.*

# TWO SIDES TO A MAN

*Sometimes when you're in a dark place, you think you've been buried but you've actually been planted*

# TWO SIDES TO A MAN

# 14.    Coping Mechanisms

Life can feel overwhelming. Having a mental breakdown or living with mental health is not easy. You might want to try different coping strategies or mechanisms to manage daily stress than you did in your past. Coping mechanisms refer to the strategies people often use in times of trauma, stress, anxiety and depression to help manage difficult or painful emotions.   Below are some coping mechanisms you might find helpful.

## **Talk with a therapist**

First rid yourself of the stigma of therapy. Working with a therapist is nothing to be shamed of, in fact, it's a luxury. Speaking with a therapist is an important element of successfully managing mental health, trauma & mental illnesses. Allowing yourself the safe space to receive therapy with a trained professional allows you to talk through any stressors and learn ways to cope with them. It's an act of self-care. Look at therapy like a sauna, but for your thoughts, a room where you can let out the steam you are harbouring in your mind.

## Express yourself in writing

What's interesting about this coping mechanism is it's actually my favourite. I tell people all the time how affective writing is in aiding mental health. Your mind is like a computer with numerous tabs open at once, and we all know how it feels to have a number of tabs open, chaotic. Well, that's how I look at the mind. Sometimes we have so much on our minds we need a place to offload them. Not everyone is comfortable with speaking about their problems to a second party, and that is also okay. But we must find ways to declutter all those tabs opened in your mind. For me I'd say the best way to tackle this is through writing. Writing is a form of therapy, self-therapy. Writing is a great method to help you manage depression and relieve stress. It enables you to be open about your thoughts, feeling and concerns without the visibility of others. Think of your favourite musicians, a lot of these guys dealt with a series of trauma and negative thoughts, but they all have one thing in common, they write it down. We listen to their songs and praise it, but these artists have found the best way to deal with their problems is to write it down and be creative with it. Now I'm not saying you have to be the next Kendrick Lamar, but what I am saying is writing is healthy, its therapy and it helps you free your mind from the clutter of your thoughts.

## Stay on the team

During difficult times, hardships and mental

health crisis, it's easy to want to retreat to a place of isolation. You must recognise that this is an avoidant coping mechanism, and it will only have a negative impact on your mental health in the long run. Instead, as I like to say, stay on the team. If you're experiencing forms of depression, you can experience a period of having low self-esteem and not wanting to be visible by the world but it's important that you push yourself. Push yourself to stay involved with your social connections and activities. Isolation corners you deeper into your thoughts, which you don't need. Don't isolate yourself from friends, family and confidants, instead use them as a crutch to save you from sinking deeper into a dark hole. Allow your confidants to take you out, have a good time and enjoy the spark of life. Don't deny yourself this luxury, you deserve to be free.

# Boost your self-image

When dealing with low points in our lives we can experience a period of low self-admiration for ourselves. We begin to not like the things we once liked, or we begin to neglect our bodies and appearance in the process. Instead of combatting a low time in your life with letting yourself go, instead do the opposite. Enhance your self-image. What better way to feel better about ourselves than feeling good about ourselves? Focusing your mind on your best qualities and accelerate them is the way to go. This can include gym or frequent haircuts to keep up with your self-care.

I mean let's not pretend when that wind hits you after you leave the barbershop you don't feel self-righteous. Let's not hide how getting that trim after a two-hour gym session makes you stay outside that little bit longer than usual. Therefore, we know that self-image helps us feel good about who we are, so during these times it's best you are nurturing exactly that.

## Stick to a schedule

If you said you're going to get up for the gym at six, get up for the gym at six. If you said you're going to put in extra hours for work, school, college, do exactly that. Sticking to a strict schedule and routine helps increase productivity which has been known to aid people with depression. I know it's difficult in times of depression as you want to spend all day in bed, not shower until the night time and feeling sorry for yourself, but you must identify that this is counterproductive.

Feeling unproductive has a way of making us feel worthless, therefore make sure you have something to do every day, even if it's as small as going for a walk, do it. It's the little things in life that give us the structure to make our day meaningful. This includes getting up, making your bed, showering early and getting out of the house for fresh air. The problem is believing you should become super productive and building houses overnight, when in fact, the aim is to increase the balance you have in your life as much as possible, one step at a time.

# TWO SIDES TO A MAN

# 15.    Conclusion

You have now made it to the end of my book, Two Sides To A Man. I hope I was able to provide some awareness of the silent battles black men are faced with and the many things which are harboured in silence. When it comes to the matters of the mind, it's safe to say it cannot be silenced, it must be expressed.

Emotions are to be explored amongst men not denied. We mustn't beat ourselves down for being unaware of these battles and how to hide them, instead we must work together actively to bring consciousness and healing. There's no better time like the present.

Made in the USA
Columbia, SC
28 January 2025

52901380R00088